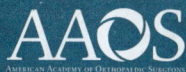

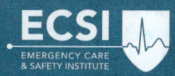

EMERGENCY CARE
& SAFETY INSTITUTE

First Aid, CPR, and AED GUIDE

EIGHTH EDITION

W0113563

Meets CPR and ECC Guidelines

American College of
Emergency Physicians®

ADVANCING EMERGENCY CARE

World Headquarters
Jones & Bartlett Learning
25 Mall Road
Burlington, MA 01803
978-443-5000
info@jblearning.com
www.jblearning.com
www.psglearning.com

Contributor Credits
Medical Writer: Alton L. Thygerson, EdD, FAWM
Medical Writer: Steven M. Thygerson, PhD, MSPH, CIH
Medical Writer: Justin S. Thygerson, PhD, CSP
Medical Editor: Alfonso Mejia, MD, MPH, FAAOS
Medical Editor: Gina Piazza, DO, FACEP
Medical Editor: Bob Elling, MPA, EMT-P

AAOS Editorial Credits
Chief Commercial Officer: Anna Salt Troise, MBA
Director, Publishing: Hans J. Koelsch, PhD
Senior Manager, Editorial: Lisa Claxton Moore
Senior Editor: Steven Kellert

Production Credits
President: Tim McClinton
VP, Product: Marisa Urbano
VP, Sales: Phil Charland
VP, Brand Strategy and Marketing: Estelle Mense
VP, Product Management: Christine Emerton
Director, Product Management: Jonathan Epstein
Product Manager: Carly Mahoney
Content Strategist: Ashley Procum
Project Manager: Kristen Rogers
Project Specialist: Madelene Nieman
Director of Sales: Brian Hendrickson

VP, International Sales: Matt Maniscalco
Director of Marketing: Brian Rooney
Production Services: Colleen Lamy
VP, Manufacturing and Inventory: Therese Connell
Composition: S4Carlisle Publishing Services
Project Management: S4Carlisle Publishing Services
Cover and Text Design: Scott Moden
Rights & Permissions Manager: John Rusk
Rights Specialist: Rebecca Damon
Senior Media Development Editor: Troy Liston
Printing and Binding: Sheridan

Library of Congress Cataloging-in-Publication Data
Library of Congress Cataloging-in-Publication Data unavailable at time of printing.

LCCN: 2019947448

6048

Printed in the United States of America
26 25   10 9 8 7 6 5

Contents

Actions to Take Before Helping

1. Size up the scene:
   - Are dangerous hazards present?
   - How many people may be in need of first aid?
   - What could be wrong with the person(s)?
   - What happened?
   - Are bystanders available to help?
2. Ask if you may help.
3. Seek professional medical care if it is needed. Depending on the seriousness and circumstances of the injury or illness, call 9-1-1 or take the person to a medical facility.
4. Protect against diseases by avoiding contact with blood and other body fluids and by washing your hands.

Injury Emergencies

Abdominal Injuries

PENETRATING OBJECT

1. **DO NOT** remove the object.
2. Stabilize the object against movement by placing bulky dressings or packing around it.
3. Call 9-1-1.

PROTRUDING (BULGING) ORGANS

1. Place the person on their back.
2. Call 9-1-1.
3. **DO NOT** try to push bulging organs back into the abdomen.

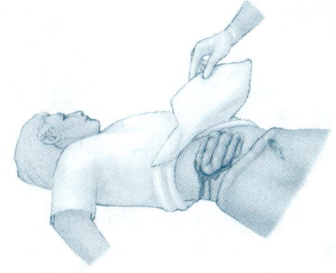

FIGURE 1 Do not reinsert protruding organs. Cover them with a moist, sterile dressing.
© Jones & Bartlett Learning.

4. Cover the wound with a sterile or clean dressing (**FIGURE 1**). Loosely tape the dressing in place. **DO NOT** apply any material that clings or disintegrates when wet.

HARD BLOW TO ABDOMEN

1. Place the person on their side with their legs bent. Be prepared for vomiting.
2. Monitor for signs of internal injuries, including the following:
    - Pain that gradually increases and may become severe
    - Pain that markedly increases with slight movements
    - Tenderness when the abdomen is touched
    - Blood in vomit or bowel movement
    - Bruising of the abdominal skin
3. Seek professional medical care if any of the preceding signs occur.

Amputations and Avulsions

AMPUTATION

1. Call 9-1-1.
2. Control bleeding by using direct pressure; if unsuccessful, apply a tourniquet or a hemostatic dressing if available.
3. Care for the amputated part (**FIGURE 2**) as follows:
   - Wrap the part in a sterile gauze or a clean cloth that has been wettened with water (make sure that excess water has been squeezed out).
   - Put the wrapped part in a waterproof container (eg, plastic bag, plastic wrap).
   - Keep the part cool by placing the container holding the part in another container with ice. **DO NOT** bury the part in the ice or allow it to touch the ice. **DO NOT** submerge it in water.
   - Send the part to the medical facility with the injured person.
4. If the amputated part was not found, ask others to search for it, and if located, to take it to the medical facility where the injured person is going.

AVULSION

An avulsion is a piece of skin that is torn loose and is hanging from the body.

1. Gently move the skin back to its normal position.
2. Cover with a sterile or clean dressing and apply pressure.
3. If bleeding continues, apply a tourniquet or a hemostatic dressing if available.

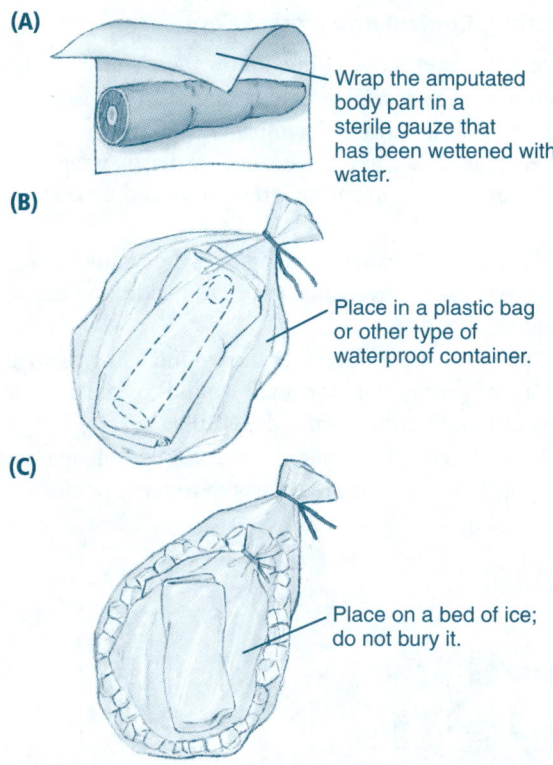

(A) Wrap the amputated body part in a sterile gauze that has been wettened with water.

(B) Place in a plastic bag or other type of waterproof container.

(C) Place on a bed of ice; do not bury it.

FIGURE 2 Care of an amputated part includes wrapping it in a sterile gauze or a clean cloth (**A**), placing it in a waterproof container (**B**), and placing it on ice (**C**).
© Jones & Bartlett Learning.

Bleeding Control and Wound Care

To care for external bleeding, follow these steps:

1. If available, wear disposable exam gloves. If exam gloves are not available, improvise a barrier (eg, plastic bag, extra dressings, or plastic wrap), or have the person apply pressure with their own hand.
2. Place a sterile gauze dressing over the wound. If a dressing is not available, use a clean cloth or your gloved hand.
3. Apply direct pressure over the wound using the flat part of your fingers for small wounds or the palm of your hand for large wounds (**FIGURE 3**).
4. If the dressing becomes blood-soaked, remove it and apply better aimed pressure with a sterile or clean dressing.

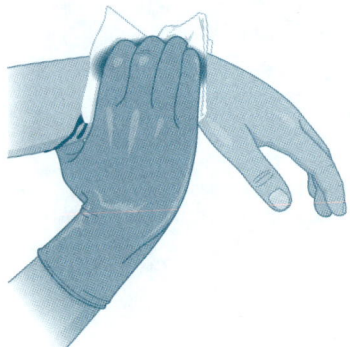

FIGURE 3 Apply direct pressure over the wound.
© Jones & Bartlett Learning.

5. If direct pressure cannot stop the bleeding:
- Call 9-1-1.
- If the bleeding is from an arm or leg, consider applying a manufactured tourniquet 2 to 3 inches (5 to 7 cm) above (proximal to) the wound and tightening it until the bleeding stops. If bleeding continues, tighten the tourniquet. If still ineffective, apply a second tourniquet near the first. A second tourniquet is rarely needed. **DO NOT** release a tourniquet. Leave a tourniquet in place until professional medical care arrives.
- Stuff a hemostatic dressing (a special dressing that helps clot the blood) into the wound if a manufactured tourniquet is not available, is ineffective, or cannot be applied (eg, wound is on the abdomen, chest, or back).
- As a last resort, improvise a tourniquet to save a life:
  - Fold a cloth into a long band about 2 to 3 inches (5 to 7 cm) wide.
  - Wrap the cloth twice around the arm or leg.
  - Tie an overhand knot
  - Place a short, rigid object (eg, screwdriver) over the overhand knot.
  - Tie a square knot over the object.
  - Twist the rigid object until bleeding stops.

When bleeding is controlled, wash your hands and care for the wound.

For a shallow wound, follow these steps:

1. Gently wash inside and around the wound with running water and with or without soap. If running

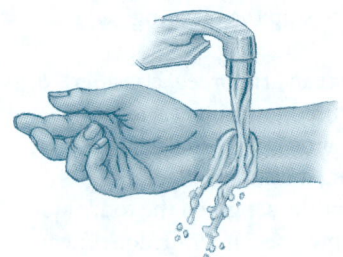

FIGURE 4 Irrigate a wound with copious amounts of water.
© Jones & Bartlett Learning.

water is not available, use any source of drinkable water.

2. Flush the wound with running water (eg, from a faucet; **FIGURE 4**). Pat the area dry with a clean cloth or towel.

3. If bleeding restarts, apply direct pressure.

4. Apply a thin layer of antibiotic ointment over the wound if the person is not sensitive to the ointment. **DO NOT** apply hydrogen peroxide, alcohol, or iodine.

5. Cover the wound with a sterile or clean dressing held in place by a bandage.

For a deep wound or a wound with a high risk of infection (eg, animal bite, very dirty or ragged wound, puncture wound), follow these steps:

1. Clean the wound. Seek professional medical care for additional wound cleaning, possible stitches, or an updated tetanus shot.

2. Cover the wound with a sterile dressing held in place by a bandage.

3. Treat for shock; keep the person from getting chilled or overheated.

Blisters

HOT SPOT

A hot spot is a painful, red area caused by rubbing.

1. Depending on availability and the blister's location, relieve pressure on the area by applying one of the following:
   - Blister bandage (eg, Blist-O-Ban)
   - Surgical tape (eg, Micropore paper tape)
   - Elastic tape (eg, Elastikon)
2. Trim and round the edges of the tape to prevent it from peeling off.

BLISTER THAT IS CLOSED AND NOT VERY PAINFUL

Depending on availability and the location of the blister, use the most appropriate method previously discussed.

BLISTER THAT IS CLOSED AND VERY PAINFUL

1. Clean the blister and a needle with an alcohol pad.
2. Make several small holes at the base of the blister with the needle (**FIGURE 5**). **DO NOT** make one large hole. Gently press the fluid out. **DO NOT** remove the blister roof unless it is torn.

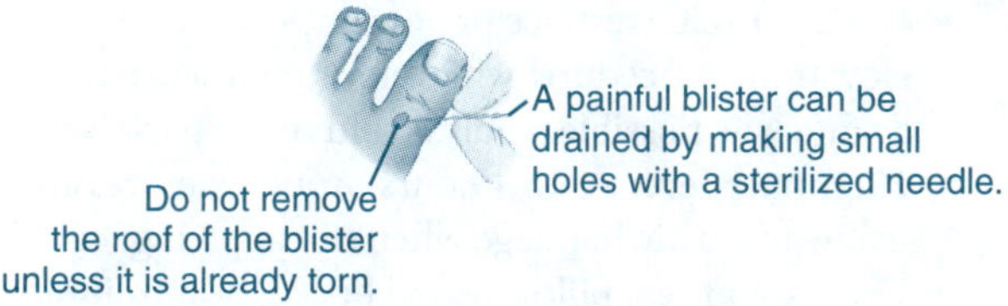

A painful blister can be drained by making small holes with a sterilized needle.

Do not remove the roof of the blister unless it is already torn.

FIGURE 5 Blister care.
© Jones & Bartlett Learning.

3. Apply paper tape to protect the blister roof from being torn away when other overlying tape is removed.
4. Cover the paper tape with elastic or adhesive tape.
5. Trim and round the edges of the tape to prevent it from peeling off.
6. Watch for signs of infection.

BLISTER THAT IS VERY PAINFUL AND OPEN OR TORN

1. Use scissors to carefully trim off the dead skin.
2. Place a blister pad (eg, Spenco 2nd Skin) over the raw skin.
3. Cover the blister pad with paper tape.
4. Cover the paper tape with elastic or adhesive tape. Trim and round the edges of the tape to prevent it from peeling off.
5. Watch for signs of infection.

Bone Injury (Broken, Fracture)

1. Hold the part when transporting a short distance to a medical facility or until arrival of emergency medical services (EMS). If EMS is delayed or if you are transporting the person a long distance, do the following:
   - Use the RICE (rest, ice pack, compression, elevation) procedure: while elevating the part as much as possible, apply a cold or ice pack for 20 minutes every 3 to 4 hours. Apply compression using an elastic bandage when not applying ice.
   - Use a splint (eg, pillow, wood board, or uninjured adjacent body part) to stabilize the part against movement (**FIGURE 6**).

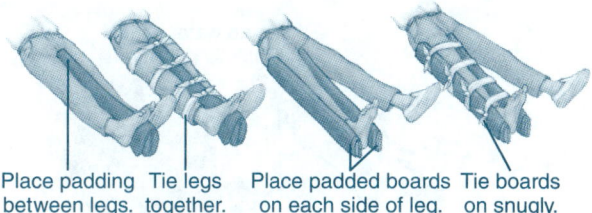

Place padding Tie legs   Place padded boards Tie boards
between legs. together.   on each side of leg. on snugly.

(A)   **(B)**

FIGURE 6 Methods of splinting leg fractures include self-splinting
(**A**) and using two boards (**B**).
© Jones & Bartlett Learning.

2. **DO NOT** move or try to straighten an injured
   extremity.
3. Call 9-1-1 for a blue or extremely pale extremity, an
   open wound, or a deformed or bent part.
4. If an open wound is bleeding, do the following:
   - Control bleeding by applying pressure to the
     wound edges. **DO NOT** push on the bone.
   - Cover the exposed bone with a sterile dressing.

Burns

THERMAL BURNS
First-Degree (Superficial) Burn
First-degree (superficial) burns are indicated by redness,
mild swelling, tenderness, and pain.
1. Immerse the burned area in cool or cold water, place
   it under running cold water, or apply a wet and cool
   or cold compress for at least 10 minutes until the

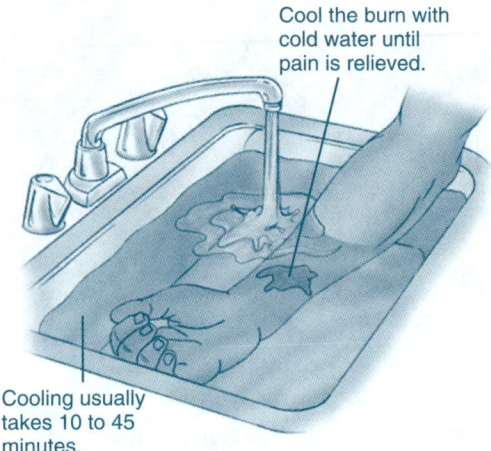

Cool the burn with cold water until pain is relieved.

Cooling usually takes 10 to 45 minutes.

FIGURE 7 Immerse the burned area in cool or cold water.
© Jones & Bartlett Learning.

pain is relieved (**FIGURE 7**). **DO NOT** apply ice, ice water, or salt water.

2. Give ibuprofen (for children and teenagers, give acetaminophen).

3. Have the person drink as much water as possible without becoming nauseous.

4. After the burn has been cooled, apply aloe vera gel or any another inexpensive skin moisturizer. First-degree burns do not need to be covered.

Small Second-Degree (Partial-Thickness) Burn

Small second-degree (partial-thickness) burns are indicated by blisters, swelling, weeping of fluids, and severe pain. To treat these burns, follow Steps 1 through 3 for first-degree burns, with the following additions:

1. After the burn has been cooled, apply a thin layer of antibacterial ointment.
2. Cover the burn with a loose, dry, nonstick, sterile or clean dressing.
3. **DO NOT** break any blisters.
4. Seek professional medical care for further advice.

Large Second-Degree (Partial-Thickness) Burn

Follow Steps 1 through 3 for first-degree burns, with the following additions:

1. Apply cold as described in Step 1 for first-degree burns, but monitor the person for hypothermia.
2. **DO NOT** break any blisters.
3. Call 9-1-1.

Third-Degree (Full-Thickness) Burn

Third-degree (full-thickness) burns are indicated by dry, leathery, gray-colored, or charred skin.

1. Cover the burn with a dry, nonstick, and sterile or clean dressing.
2. **DO NOT** apply gel or ointment to the burn.
3. **DO NOT** apply cold.
4. Call 9-1-1.

ELECTRICAL BURNS

1. If the person is inside a building and in contact with electricity, turn off the electricity or unplug the appliance.

2. If the person is in contact with an outdoor power line, call 9-1-1 to have the electricity turned off or wires cut.
3. **DO NOT** touch or move the person or the electrical wires or appliances (even with a wooden pole, rope, or any other item).
4. Keep people away from the area.
5. Call 9-1-1 immediately. Every person who has been electrocuted needs professional medical care.
6. Once the area is safe:
   - Check the breathing of any unresponsive person; if absent, begin cardiopulmonary resuscitation (CPR). If the person is breathing, place them on their side.
   - Loosely cover the burn with a dry, sterile dressing. **DO NOT** apply gel or ointment to the burn.

CHEMICAL BURNS

First aid is the same for most chemical burns.

1. Call 9-1-1 immediately for all chemical burns.
2. If the burn occurred at a workplace, send someone to check the safety data sheet (SDS) for hazardous materials used at the work site.
3. Once the area is safe, brush any dry or powder chemical off the skin with a gloved hand or piece of cloth before flushing with water.
4. Flush the burn immediately with large amounts of cold running water for at least 20 minutes or until EMS arrives (**FIGURE 8**). Clothing or jewelry that covers the burn area can be removed.
5. **DO NOT** try to neutralize the chemical.

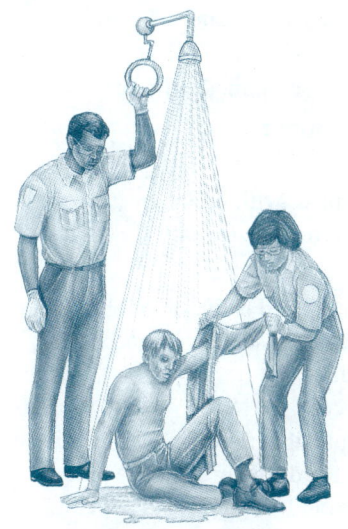

FIGURE 8 Flushing a chemical burn.
© Jones & Bartlett Learning.

6. If an eye is affected, tip the head so the affected eye is below the nose, and wash the eye with warm water from the nose out to the side of the face for at least 15 to 20 minutes. If both eyes are affected, wash them with warm water at the same time.

Chest Injuries

RIB FRACTURES

1. Stabilize the chest by either of the following methods:
   - Have the person hold a pillow or other similarly soft material against the area.
   - Place the arm on the injured side in a sling and binder.

2. **DO NOT** apply tight bandages around the chest.
3. Give pain medication.
4. Call 9-1-1 or seek professional medical care.

PENETRATING (IMPALED) OBJECT
1. Call 9-1-1.
2. Stabilize the object in place with bulky dressings or padding. **DO NOT** try to remove the object.

OPEN CHEST WOUND
Open chest wounds are indicated by blood bubbling out of the chest during exhalation, a sucking sound heard during inhalation, or both.
1. If bleeding does not occur, **DO NOT** cover the wound.
2. If bleeding occurs, apply direct pressure with a dry gauze dressing. If the dressing becomes blood-soaked, replace it to avoid trapping air in the chest, which can result in death.
3. Call 9-1-1.

Ear Injuries

OBJECT STUCK IN THE EAR
1. **DO NOT** use tweezers or try to pry the object out.
2. Seek professional medical care to remove the object. Except for disc batteries and live insects, few foreign bodies must be removed immediately.

FLUIDS COMING FROM THE EAR
Blood or clear fluid coming from the ear may indicate a skull fracture.
1. **DO NOT** attempt to stop the flow of blood or clear fluid (with or without blood) coming from an ear.

2. Loosely bandage a sterile gauze dressing over the ear.
3. Stabilize the head and neck against movement. Tell the person to remain as still as possible.
4. Call 9-1-1.

Impaled (Embedded) Object

This section covers treatment to be followed when a large object, such as a nail, knife, or steel rod, is stuck in the body.

1. **DO NOT** remove or move the object.
2. Stabilize the object with bulky dressings or padding placed around the base of the object to keep it from moving.
3. If the wound site is bleeding, apply direct pressure around the base of the object. **DO NOT** apply pressure on the object or on the skin next to the sharp edges of the object.
4. Call 9-1-1.

Eye Injuries

BLOW TO EYE

1. Apply an ice pack around the eye for 15 minutes. **DO NOT** place the ice pack on the eye.
2. Have the person keep both eyes closed.
3. Seek professional medical care.

LOOSE OBJECT IN EYE

Try, in order, each of the following steps:

1. Have the person blink the eye several times.
2. Using the eyelashes, pull the upper eyelid out and over the lower lid.

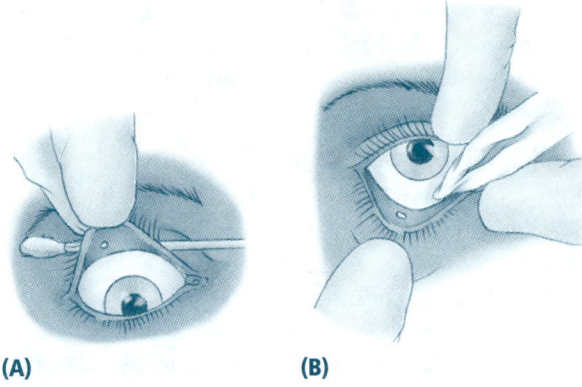

(A)   **(B)**

FIGURE 9 A. To remove a foreign object from the eye, lift the upper eyelid up and over a cotton swab. **B**. Examine the lower lid by gently pulling it down. If an object is seen, remove it with a wet gauze pad.
© Jones & Bartlett Learning.

3. Examine the lower lid by pulling it down gently.
4. Gently irrigate the eye with clean, warm water.
5. Lift the upper eyelid up and over a cotton swab. If the object is seen, remove it with the corner of a wet gauze pad (**FIGURE 9**).
6. If any of the previously discussed methods are successful, professional medical care is usually not needed unless there is continued pain or itching in the eye.

OBJECT STUCK IN EYE

1. **DO NOT** remove the object.
2. For a long object, place padding around it to stabilize against movement.

3. For a short object, place a doughnut-shaped pad around the eye and wrap a bandage around the head to hold the pad in place.
4. Cover both eyes; movement of the uninjured eye will cause movement of the injured eye, which could cause more damage.
5. Keep the person flat on their back.
6. Call 9-1-1 as soon as possible.

CHEMICAL, SMOKE, OR OTHER IRRITANT IN EYE

1. Hold the eye wide open and flush with warm water, normal saline, or other eye irrigation solution for at least 15 minutes. Tip the head so the eye is below the nose and flush from the nose out to the side of the face to avoid having the chemical run into the unaffected eye (**FIGURE 10**).

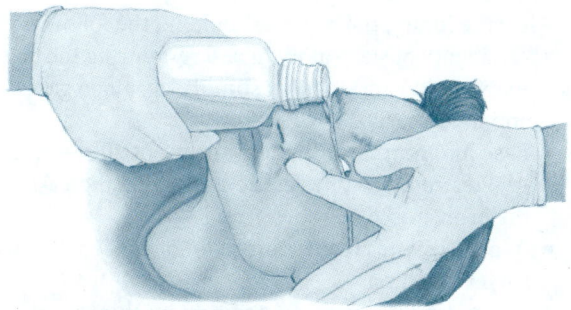

FIGURE 10 Immediately flush the eye in cases of chemical injuries.
© Jones & Bartlett Learning.

2. Call 9-1-1 and continue flushing with warm water until EMS arrives.
3. Loosely bandage the eye.

Head Injuries

BRAIN INJURY (CONCUSSION)

A concussion is a brain injury occurring when the brain moves inside the skull from a sudden head movement or blow to the head. Recognizing a concussion is difficult.

1. If the person is unresponsive, check for breathing; if absent, call 9-1-1 and give CPR.
2. If a neck or spinal injury is suspected, do the following:
   - **DO NOT** move the head, neck, or spine.
   - Tell the person to remain as still as possible.
   - Call 9-1-1.
3. When in doubt about the person's condition, seek professional medical care as soon as possible.
4. After the injury, the person should do the following:
   - Get plenty of sleep at night and rest during the day.
   - Avoid visual and sensory stimuli (eg, video games and loud music).
   - Ease into normal activities slowly, not all at once.
   - Avoid strenuous physical activities that increase the heart rate.
   - Avoid activities that require a lot of concentration, such as reading.
   - Avoid driving, cycling, operating machinery, or playing sports until approved by a health care provider.

- Avoid anything that could cause another blow to the head or body.
- **DO NOT** use aspirin or anti-inflammatory medications (ie, ibuprofen) because of the risk of bleeding. Acetaminophen can be used for postconcussion headaches.

SCALP WOUND

1. Control bleeding by pressing on the wound. Replace any skin flap to its original position and apply pressure. For a bruise without external bleeding, apply an ice pack or instant cold pack.
2. Apply a dry, sterile or clean dressing.
3. Keep the head and shoulders raised if no spinal injury is suspected.
4. If the dressing becomes blood-soaked, remove it and apply better aimed pressure with a clean dressing.
5. Call 9-1-1 if:
   - The wound is extensive.
   - Significant facial damage is present.
   - Signs of concussion occur (eg, nausea and vomiting, headache, drowsiness).

SKULL FRACTURE

A skull fracture may be indicated by skull deformity; blood or clear, watery fluid coming from an ear or the nose; unequal-sized pupils; and heavy scalp bleeding.

1. Apply a sterile or clean dressing over the wound and hold it in place with gentle pressure.

2. Control bleeding by pressing on the edges of the wound.
3. Call 9-1-1.
4. *Cautions:*
   - **DO NOT** move the head, neck, or spine.
   - **DO NOT** clean the wound.
   - **DO NOT** remove an embedded object.
   - **DO NOT** stop blood or clear fluid that is draining from an ear or the nose.
   - **DO NOT** press on the fractured area.

Joint Injuries

DISLOCATION

A dislocation occurs when a joint comes apart and stays apart.

1. Call 9-1-1 for a blue or extremely pale extremity, an open wound, or a deformed or bent part.
2. Hold the part still when transporting the person a short distance to a medical facility or, if 9-1-1 has been called, until EMS arrives.
3. If EMS is delayed or if you are transporting the person a long distance, do the following:
   - Use the RICE procedure (rest, ice pack, compression, elevation).
   - Use a splint (eg, pillow, wood board, or uninjured adjacent body part) to stabilize the part against movement.
4. **DO NOT** move or try to reset an injured extremity.

5. If an open wound is bleeding, do the following:
- Control the bleeding by applying pressure to the wound edges.
- **DO NOT** push on the bone.

SPRAIN
A sprain occurs when the joint's ligaments are stretched and injured.

1. Most sprains do not require professional medical care. If recuperation seems long, consult a physician.

2. Use the RICE procedure (rest, ice pack, compression, elevation).

Muscle Injuries

BRUISE
A bruise is an injury, usually caused by a blow to the area, that causes bleeding beneath the skin without breaking the skin.

Use the RICE procedure (rest, ice pack, compression, elevation).

CRAMP
A cramp is a sudden, often painful muscle contraction or spasm.

1. Try one or more of the following methods to relax the muscle:
- Gently stretch the affected muscle.
- Press on the muscle.
- Apply an ice pack to the muscle.

- If cramping occurs during exertion in a hot environment, drink lightly salted, cool water (dissolve one-fourth teaspoon [1.25 mL] salt in 1 quart [about 1 L] of water) or a commercial sports drink.
2. **DO NOT** give salt tablets.

STRAIN

A strain is the stretching or tearing of a muscle; this injury is also called a "muscle pull".

Use the RICE procedure (rest, ice pack, compression, elevate).

Nosebleed

1. If the nose was hit, suspect a broken nose.
2. Have the person sit leaning slightly forward (**FIGURE 11**). **DO NOT** tilt the head back or lay the person down.
3. Pinch the nostrils shut constantly for 10 minutes. Tell the person to breathe through the mouth and not swallow any blood.
4. If the bleeding has not stopped by that time, have the person gently sniff or blow their nose to get rid of ineffective blood clots. Pinch the nostrils together again for 10 minutes.
5. Professional medical care is not usually needed unless bleeding continues, a foreign object is in the nose, or the nose is broken.

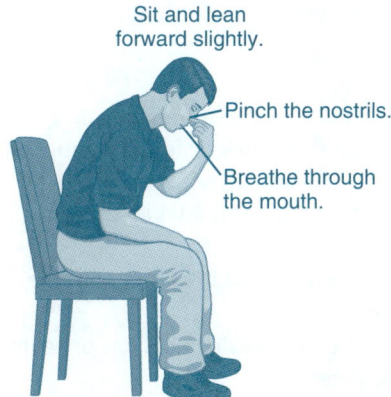

Sit and lean
forward slightly.

Pinch the nostrils.

Breathe through
the mouth.

FIGURE 11
Positioning of a person
pinching the nostrils to
stop a nosebleed.
© Jones & Bartlett Learning.

Shock

Shock can happen when a large amount of blood loss
occurs. Do not confuse this condition with an electrical
shock or being "shocked," as in scared or surprised.
Shock is life threatening. Expect and treat for shock if a
person has any of the following conditions:

- Massive external or internal bleeding
- Severe infection
- Broken bones
- Heart attack
- Abdominal or chest injury
- Severe allergic reaction

Even if there are no signs of shock (ie, anxiety and
restlessness; pale, cool, and moist skin; rapid breathing

and heartbeat; nausea or vomiting), you should still do the following:

1. Treat injuries.
2. If the person is responsive and breathing normally, keep the person flat on their back. Another option is to raise the feet 6 to 12 inches (15 to 30 cm), if there is no sign of a leg injury and doing so does not cause pain (**FIGURE 12**).
3. If the person is unresponsive and breathing, roll the person onto their side.
4. Prevent loss of body heat by putting blankets or coats under and over the person.
5. Call 9-1-1.
6. **DO NOT** give anything to eat or drink unless professional medical help is delayed for over 1 hour, in which case sips of water can be given.
7. Monitor breathing; if absent, give CPR.

Spinal Injury

1. Suspect a spinal injury whenever:
    - One of the following mechanisms of injury is involved:
        - A motor vehicle crash involving ejection, a rollover, high speeds, or pedestrians
        - Other types of motorized vehicle crash (eg, motorcycle, scooter, all-terrain vehicle, snowmobile)
        - A bicycle or skateboard crash
        - A fall greater than the person's standing height, especially if the person is older

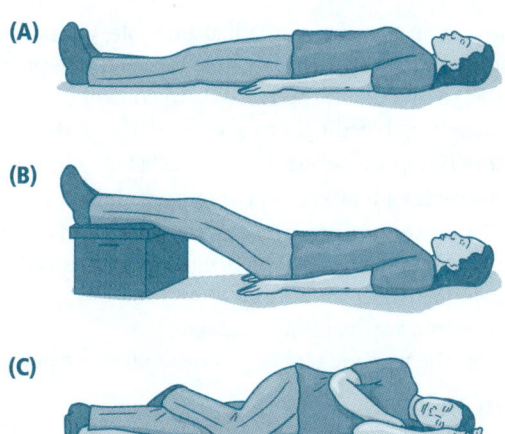

FIGURE 12 Shock positions. **A**. If the person is responsive and breathing normally, keep the person flat on their back. **B**. If there is no sign of injury and doing so does not cause pain, feet can be raised 6 to 12 inches (15 to 30 cm). **C**. If the person is unresponsive and breathing normally, roll the person onto their side.
© Jones & Bartlett Learning.

- - A dive into shallow water
  - A hit or blow to the head
  - The person complains of back pain, leg numbness, and tingling
  - The person cannot (a) wiggle their toes or fingers and cannot (b) identify which toe or finger is pinched when their eyes are closed
2. Given any of these scenarios, call 9-1-1.
3. **DO NOT** attempt to move the person. Leave the person in the position in which they were found. Tell

the person to remain as still as possible. Consider moving the person only for the following: to provide CPR, to open a blocked airway, to control life-threatening bleeding, or to reach a safe location.

4. **DO NOT** apply a cervical (neck) collar.
5. Cover with a blanket or coat to prevent heat loss.
6. If the person is unresponsive, has an altered mental status, or is intoxicated by drugs and/or alcohol, do the following:
   - Assume a spinal injury exists.
   - Use the methods in Step 3 to stabilize the person.

Mouth Bleeding

1. Allow blood to drain out of the mouth.
2. For a bleeding tongue, put a dressing on the wound and apply pressure.
3. For a cut through a lip, place a rolled gauze dressing between the lip and the gum and press another dressing against the outer lip.
4. Transport the person to professional medical care if bleeding continues or stitches are needed.

Tooth Injuries

KNOCKED-OUT TOOTH

This section applies only to adult, or permanent, teeth.

1. Seek a dentist immediately.
2. Take the tooth to the dentist. **DO NOT** let the tooth dry out. For that purpose, store the tooth in one of the following solutions (listed in order of preference):

- Hank's Balanced Salt Solution (eg, Save-A-Tooth)
- Clear plastic wrap
- Cow's milk (any percent fat is OK)
- The person's saliva spit into a small container, if available. **DO NOT** store the tooth in the mouth, in water, or in your or another person's saliva.

3. If the person is unable to see a dentist within an hour of the injury, attempt to put the tooth back in its socket as follows:
   - Hold the tooth by the crown. **DO NOT** touch the root.
   - Rinse the tooth in a bowl of warm water. **DO NOT** scrub or touch the root.
   - Gently push the tooth into the socket so that the top is even with the adjacent teeth. The person can bite down gently on gauze or cloth placed between the teeth.

BROKEN TOOTH

1. Collect the tooth or teeth fragments and store them in any of the solutions that you would use for a knocked-out tooth.
2. Seek a dentist as soon as possible; the dentist may be able to reattach the broken pieces.
3. Keep the mouth closed to reduce pain.

LOOSENED TOOTH

1. Cover the tooth with a piece of gauze or cloth and bite down to keep it in place.
2. Consult a dentist.

Sudden Illnesses

Allergic Reactions (Severe)

Severe allergic reaction (anaphylaxis) may be indicated by shortness of breath; swelling of the lips, tongue, mouth, nose, and throat; intense itching of the skin and throat; flushed skin or swollen face; trouble swallowing, breathing, coughing, or wheezing; cramps, nausea, or vomiting; or a medical identification tag indicating an allergy.

1. Call 9-1-1.
2. Monitor breathing; if absent, give CPR.
3. If the person has their own medically prescribed epinephrine auto-injector, you may need to get it and help the person self-administer it. If the person is not capable of using it and you are allowed by state law to give an injection, use the person's prescribed epinephrine auto-injector as follows:
   a. Find the injection site on the outer midthigh between the knee and the hip. Check for coins, keys, and pant seams, which could obstruct the needle.
   b. Remove the safety cap. Hold the auto-injector in your fist without touching either end of the pen.
   c. Push the auto-injector until you hear a click against the outer midthigh (if necessary, the injection can be done through light clothing).
   d. Hold in place for 3 seconds.
   e. Pull the auto-injector straight out from the leg.

    f. Rub the area for 10 seconds.

    g. Put the auto-injector back into its safety case.

4. If the first dose does not help and EMS arrival will exceed 5 to 10 minutes, consider giving a second dose.

Asthma

Asthma causes breathing difficulty. This condition varies from one person to another and can be life threatening.

1. Place the person in an upright sitting position, leaning slightly forward.

2. Encourage the person to sit quietly and breathe slowly and deeply in through the nose and out through the mouth.

3. Ask the person about any asthma medication they use. Most people with asthma have a physician-prescribed quick-relief (rescue) inhaler with a spacer or holding chamber.

4. Help the person use their quick-relief inhaler as follows:

    a. Remove the cap and shake the inhaler vigorously 10 to 15 times. Apply the spacer, if available.

    b. For greater benefit, the person can take a breath without the inhaler and then breathe all the way out.

    c. Hold the inhaler upright (or have the person do so if they can). Tell the person to place their lips around the inhaler or spacer. If using a spacer, have the person wait 5 seconds before breathing in.

    d. Have the person start breathing in slowly and then press down on the inhaler once while breathing in all the air they can. Then tell them to hold their breath for 10 seconds. If using a spacer, have the person wait 5 seconds before breathing in.

    e. When the 10 seconds is up, tell the person to open their mouth and breathe out slowly.

    f. A second dose may be given in 30 to 60 seconds. **DO NOT** exceed the prescribed dose.

5. Call 9-1-1 immediately if:

- The person is struggling to breathe, talk, or stay awake.
- They are unable to speak more than one to two words in one breath.
- Their lips or fingernails turn blue or gray.
- The person asks for professional medical care.
- There is no improvement after using the medication.
- Repeated attacks occur.
- A severe and prolonged attack occurs.

Choking

To provide care for an airway obstruction, refer to pages 64–69.

Diabetic Emergencies

HYPOGLYCEMIA (BLOOD SUGAR TOO LOW)

Hypoglycemia (low blood glucose) is a life-threatening emergency that occurs when a person with diabetes does one of the following:

- Takes too much insulin (rapidly depletes sugar)

- Does not eat enough food or vomits (reduces sugar intake)
- Does more physical activity than usual (uses sugar faster)

If the person is responsive, alert, and can swallow, they may be able to tell you what to do.

1. If the person has a blood glucose monitor, allow them to check their blood glucose.
2. If testing is not possible, testing shows a low blood sugar level (below 70 mg/dL), or profuse sweating or shaking occurs in a person known to have diabetes, then follow these steps:
   a. Have the person eat 15 to 20 grams of sugar (8 to 10 grams for children).
   b. If available, 3 to 5 glucose tablets is preferred. If glucose tablets are not available, give the person any form of sugar, such as glucose gel as directed on the label, 4 ounces (one-half cup) of fruit juice or regular soda (not diet), 3 to 5 teaspoons of table sugar or honey, hard candies, jellybeans, or other sugary food (check the label to determine how much to give).
   c. Wait 10 to 15 minutes for the sugar to get into the blood.
   d. Recheck the blood glucose level, or if there is no monitor, check the person for improvement. If it is still low or no monitor was used and the person still has symptoms of low blood sugar, give the person 15 more grams of sugar.

3. If there is still no improvement, call 9-1-1 as soon as possible.

If the person is unresponsive, unable to follow simple instructions, or unable to swallow:

1. Call 9-1-1 immediately.
2. Monitor breathing; if absent, give CPR.
3. Look for a medical identification tag.
4. **DO NOT** give any food or drink.
5. Place the person on their side to keep the airway open and to drain fluids or vomit from the mouth.

HYPERGLYCEMIA (BLOOD SUGAR TOO HIGH)

Hyperglycemia (high blood glucose) occurs when a person with diabetes has too much sugar in their blood. Several conditions can cause hyperglycemia (eg, insufficient insulin, overeating, illness, inactivity, stress, or a combination of these factors). Most people with diabetes can recognize what is happening and will adjust their insulin dose or seek professional medical help before serious problems develop; however, if it is not treated within 24 hours, hyperglycemia can be fatal.

1. Give frequent, small sips of water if the person with diabetes can swallow.
2. If uncertain whether the person with diabetes has a high or low blood glucose level, and if they are responsive and able to swallow, use the rules for giving sugar as previously described. The extra sugar will not cause significant harm in a person experiencing hyperglycemia.

3. **DO NOT** give insulin unless the person with diabetes can self-administer it.
4. Call 9-1-1 as soon as possible.

Fainting

If a person has already fainted, do the following:

1. Check breathing; if the person is not breathing or is only occasionally gasping, call 9-1-1, get an automated external defibrillator (AED), and give CPR.
2. If the person is breathing:
   - Keep the person flat on their back. Their feet can be raised 6 to 12 inches (15 to 30 cm) if doing so does not cause pain.
   - Monitor breathing; if the person stops breathing or is only occasionally gasping, call 9-1-1 and give CPR.
   - Loosen tight clothing.
   - If the person fell, check and treat any injuries.
   - Wipe the person's forehead with a cool, wet cloth.
   - **DO NOT** use ammonia inhalants or smelling salts.
   - **DO NOT** give the person anything to drink or eat until they have fully recovered and can swallow.
   - **DO NOT** splash or pour water on the person's face.
   - **DO NOT** slap the person's face in an attempt to revive them.
3. Call 9-1-1 if:
   - Repeated episodes occur.
   - The person does not regain responsiveness quickly.

- The person has diabetes, has seizures, is pregnant, has a loss of bowel or bladder control, is older than 50 years, or has no obvious reason for fainting.

Heart Attack

A heart attack may be indicated by pain in the chest, arms, or neck; shortness of breath; dizziness; or fainting.

1. Have the person sit, with knees raised, and lean against a stable but comfortable support. Try to keep the person calm. **DO NOT** allow the person to walk.
2. Call 9-1-1 immediately. **DO NOT** transport the person to a medical facility; wait for EMS to arrive.
3. While waiting for EMS to arrive, do the following:
   - Loosen any tight clothing.
   - Ask if the person takes any chest pain medication, such as nitroglycerin, for a known heart condition, and if so, help them take it if they can.
   - If the person is alert, is able to swallow, is not allergic to aspirin, and has no signs of stroke, help the person to take one adult aspirin (325 mg) or two to four low-dose aspirins (81 mg each). Pulverize or have the person chew the pill or pills before swallowing for faster results.
   - Monitor breathing. If the person becomes unresponsive and stops breathing, begin CPR. If they are unresponsive and are breathing, place them on their side.

Hyperventilation

Hyperventilation is fast breathing (more than 40 breaths per minute) during emotional distress.

1. Calm and reassure the person.
2. Take the person to a quiet place or ask bystanders to leave. Have the person sit down.
3. Encourage the person to breathe slowly and to inhale through the nose, hold the inhalation for 1 to 2 seconds, and then exhale slowly through pursed lips.
4. Ask the person about physician-prescribed medication for the condition and help them take it if available and they desire it.

Pregnancy Complications

SEVERE STOMACH PAIN OR CRAMPS

Short, mild cramps near the delivery date may be normal; the woman may be in labor if the cramps are strong and repetitive or her water has broken. If pain persists or labor is suspected, seek immediate professional medical care.

SEIZURE

Seizures during pregnancy may indicate a serious complication.

1. Provide appropriate care for seizures (see pages 40–41).
2. Call 9-1-1 immediately.

VAGINAL BLEEDING

1. Have the woman place a sanitary pad or a towel to absorb the blood. **DO NOT** pack the vagina.
2. Call 9-1-1 immediately.

SUDDEN LEAKAGE OF FLUID

A sudden leakage of fluid may indicate the beginning of labor. Seek immediate professional medical care.

MORNING SICKNESS

1. Treat nausea and vomiting by giving the woman small amounts of clear fluids (eg, sports drinks, apple juice) to drink. If the woman is able to keep down fluids, offer her bread or cereal.
2. Have the woman rest.
3. If vomiting persists, seek professional medical care.

Seizure

A seizure may be indicated by the person suddenly collapsing, becoming unresponsive, and having spasms or convulsions.

1. Move nearby objects to avoid injury to the person. Place something soft (eg, a rolled towel) under the person's head. **DO NOT** use a pillow.
2. **DO NOT** try to hold the person down.
3. **DO NOT** put anything between the person's teeth or give anything by mouth.
4. Time the seizure from start to finish.
5. Most seizures do not require calling 9-1-1 and end in 1 to 2 minutes.
6. Call 9-1-1 for any of the following:
   - A seizure lasting longer than 5 minutes
   - A series of seizures following one another
   - Breathing difficulties
   - A seizure that happens in water

- This is the person's first known seizure
- The person is injured or pregnant or has diabetes
- Slow recovery
- The person asks for professional medical help

7. After the seizure, do the following:
   - Monitor breathing; if absent, call 9-1-1, get an AED, and give CPR.
   - Allow the person to sleep.
   - Keep the airway open by placing the person on their side.
   - Stay with the person until they are alert.

Stroke

Identify the common signs of a stroke by using the **FAST** mnemonic.

- **F = Face droops**: Ask the person to smile. Does one side of the face droop?
- **A = Arm weakness**: Ask the person to close their eyes and raise both arms with the palms up. Does one arm drift downward?
- **S = Speech difficulty**: Ask the person to repeat a simple phrase or sentence (eg, "the sky is blue"). Does the person slur their speech or use the wrong words, or are they unable to speak at all?
- **T = Time to call**: Call 9-1-1 immediately if any of the signs previously discussed occur.

If the person displays signs of a stroke do the following:

1. Call 9-1-1.

2. Monitor responsiveness and breathing:
   - If the person is unresponsive and not breathing, begin CPR.
   - If they are unresponsive and breathing or have fluid or vomit in their mouth, place them on their side (the recovery position).
   - If they are alert, allow them to find a comfortable position with the head and shoulders above the body.
3. **DO NOT** give the person anything to eat or drink.

Environmental Emergencies

Bites and Stings

ANIMAL BITES

1. **DO NOT** try to capture the animal. Instead, try to remember its description and last location so that authorities can find and manage the animal.
2. **DO NOT** kill the animal. If you think that you must kill a wild animal, **DO NOT** hit or shoot its head (brain). Though often impossible, the animal's brain can be tested for the rabies virus.
3. Contact the local health department.

BITE THAT HAS BROKEN THE SKIN

1. Stop the bleeding by applying direct pressure over the wound.
2. Wash inside and around the wound with soap and running water.

3. Flush the inside of the wound with clean running water.
4. If bleeding reoccurs, reapply direct pressure over the wound. Once the bleeding stops, apply a thin layer of an over-the-counter (OTC) antibiotic ointment and cover the wound with a sterile dressing.
5. For all bites that break the skin, transport the person to a medical facility, where providers will do the following:
   - Clean the wound.
   - Close wide and gaping open wounds.
   - Administer a tetanus booster, if necessary.

BITE THAT HAS NOT BROKEN THE SKIN
Apply an ice pack for up to 20 minutes, placing a paper towel or thin, damp cloth between the skin and the ice pack.

INSECT STINGS
1. If a stinger is found, immediately scrape it off the skin with a fingernail or plastic card (eg, credit card) or brush it off with your hand.
2. Wash the area with soap and running water.
3. Apply an ice pack for up to 20 minutes, placing a paper towel or thin cloth between the skin and the ice pack.
4. To relieve itching and swelling, apply hydrocortisone cream (1%) and give the person an antihistamine.
5. For a severe allergic reaction that could be life threatening, help the person self-administer their physician-prescribed epinephrine (see pages 32–33).

6. Monitor breathing; if absent, call 9-1-1 and give CPR.
7. For a sting in the mouth or throat, have the person suck on ice unless swelling causes breathing difficulty (in that case, call 9-1-1).

SNAKE BITES

1. Get the person and bystanders away from the snake. A dead snake can still bite, even if decapitated.
2. Encourage the person to rest, stay calm, and be still.
3. **DO NOT** try to capture or kill the snake. Try to remember the snake's color and the shape of its head. Taking a clear photograph from a safe distance (ie, more than the length of the snake) can help with identifying the snake.
4. Remove any rings, jewelry, or tight clothing from the bitten body part to avoid blood constriction from swelling.
5. Gently wash the bite with soap and running water, and apply a sterile dressing over the fang marks.
6. Call 9-1-1 or transport the person to a medical facility as soon as possible.

Pit Vipers

Pit vipers include rattlesnakes, copperheads, and cottonmouths (ie, water moccasins; **FIGURE 13**).

1. When possible, carry the person. If the person is alone and capable, they should walk slowly.
2. *Cautions:*
   - **DO NOT** apply a pressure bandage.

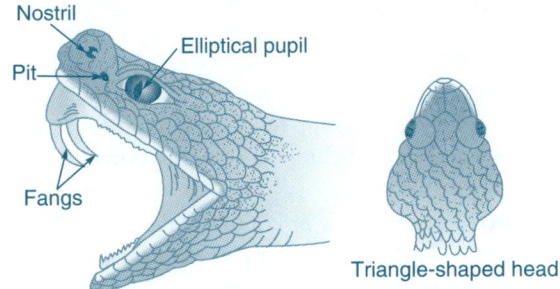

FIGURE 13 Characteristic features of pit vipers.
© Jones & Bartlett Learning.

- **DO NOT** cut the person's skin to drain the venom.
- **DO NOT** use mouth suction or any suction device to try to remove the venom.
- **DO NOT** apply cold packs or ice packs.
- **DO NOT** give alcohol.
- **DO NOT** apply electrical shock.
- **DO NOT** use a tourniquet.

CORAL SNAKES

1. Apply a wide elastic bandage using overlapping turns. Start wrapping at the end of the bitten arm or leg and wrap upward, covering its entire length.
2. Adhere to the cautions previously given for pit vipers, except that pressure bandages can be used.

NONVENOMOUS SNAKES

1. Treat the bite the same as you would a shallow wound, as described on pages 9–10.

2. Consult a physician.

SPIDER BITES

1. Wash the bite site with soap and running water.
2. Apply an ice pack for up to 20 minutes, placing a paper towel or thin cloth between the skin and the ice pack.
3. **DO NOT** try to capture or kill the spider. Try to remember the spider's color and markings. Taking a clear photograph from a safe distance can help with identifying the spider.
4. Seek professional medical care as soon as possible.

TICK (EMBEDDED)

To remove the tick, follow these steps:

1. Use tweezers or a specialized tick-removal tool to grasp the tick as close to the person's skin as possible (**FIGURE 14**).

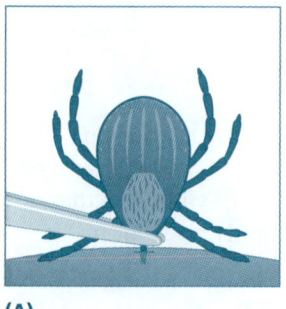 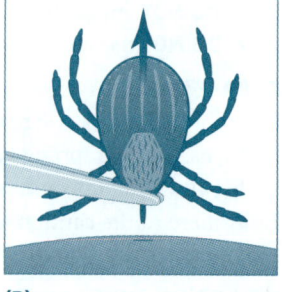

(A)   **(B)**

FIGURE 14 Tick removal with tweezers: **A**. Grasp the tick. **B**. Pull upward.

2. Pull upward with steady, even pressure to tent the skin surface. Hold in this position until the tick lets go (up to 1 minute). **DO NOT** twist or jerk the tick.

3. **DO NOT** use any of the following ineffective methods to remove the tick:
   - Petroleum jelly
   - Fingernail polish
   - Rubbing alcohol
   - Gasoline
   - Touching with a blown-out hot match, hot needle, or hot paper clip

4. **DO NOT** grab a tick at the rear of its body; the tick's internal contents could be squeezed into the person.

When the tick is completely removed, follow these steps:

1. Wash your hands and the wound area with soap and running water. Apply rubbing alcohol to further disinfect the area.

2. Apply an ice pack for up to 20 minutes, placing a paper towel or thin cloth between the skin and the ice pack.

3. Apply calamine lotion or 1% hydrocortisone cream to relieve itching.

4. Place the tick in a plastic bag and bring it to a physician for identification if the person needs professional medical care (see Step 5).

5. If a rash, fever, or flulike symptoms (headache, body aches, and/or nausea) occur within 3 to 30 days of

the tick's removal, seek professional medical care—
with or without the tick.

Cold-Related Emergencies

FROSTBITE

Frostbite occurs only in below-freezing temperatures
(less than 32°F [0°C]).

1. Move the person to a warm place.
2. Remove any wet clothing and constricting items,
   such as rings, that could impair blood circulation.
3. Use the following wet, rapid rewarming method if
   (a) professional medical care is more than 2 hours
   away, (b) there is no possibility of refreezing the
   affected area, and (c) shelter, warm water, and a
   container are available: Place the frostbitten part in
   warm (100°F to 104°F [38°C to 40°C]) water. If you
   do not have a thermometer, put your hand into the
   water to test that it will not burn. For ear or facial
   injuries, apply warm, moist cloths, changing them
   frequently. Allow slow thawing (thawing in a warm
   room without warm water or warm cloths) of a part
   if it is the only method available.
4. *Cautions:*
   - **DO NOT** rub or massage the affected area.
   - **DO NOT** apply ice, snow, or cold water to the
     affected area.
   - **DO NOT** rewarm the affected area with a stove or
     over a fire.
   - **DO NOT** break blisters.

- **DO NOT** allow the thawed part to refreeze, as this will cause greater damage.

After thawing, follow these steps:

1. If the feet are affected, **DO NOT** allow the person to walk.
2. Protect the injured area from contact with clothing and bedding.
3. Apply aloe vera gel to promote skin healing.
4. Place bulky, dry, clean gauze on the affected part and between the toes/fingers to absorb moisture and keep them from sticking together.
5. Give ibuprofen to limit pain and inflammation.
6. Seek professional medical care as soon as possible.

Cold Stress

Cold stress occurs when the body's temperature drops. The symptoms are not as severe as those with hypothermia.

1. If the person's clothing is wet, allow the person to remove them.
2. Give high-calorie food or drink.
3. Have them move about and exercise to warm up.
4. Consider using a warm shower or bath.

HYPOTHERMIA

Hypothermia does not require subfreezing temperatures.

1. Stop the heat loss by doing the following:
   a. Move the person to a warm place. Handle the person very gently.

   b.   Replace wet clothing with dry clothing.
   c.   Add insulation (eg, blankets, towels) beneath
           and around the person. Cover the person's
           head.
   d.   Cover the person with a vapor barrier (eg, a
           tarp, trash bags) to prevent heat loss. If unable
           to remove wet clothing, place a vapor barrier
           between the clothing and the insulation. For
           a person who is dry, the vapor barrier can be
           placed outside the insulation.
2.   Keep the person in a flat (horizontal) position.
3.   Call 9-1-1.
4.   If possible, apply heat to the person's armpits, chest,
        and back (in that order). Use large electric pads or
        blankets, large chemical heat pads, or warm water
        bottles. Place insulation between the skin and the
        heat source to prevent burning the skin.

Mild Hypothermia

Mild hypothermia may be indicated by vigorous,
uncontrollable shivering; the "umbles" (grumbles,
mumbles, fumbles, stumbles, and tumbles); or cool or
cold skin on the abdomen, chest, or back. In addition to
the previously discussed steps for treating a person with
hypothermia, do the following:

1.   Give warm, sugary drinks. **DO NOT** give the person
        alcohol.
2.   If the person is adequately rewarmed and has a
        normal mental status, they will usually not need to
        be transported to professional medical care.

Severe Hypothermia

Severe hypothermia may be indicated by rigid and stiff muscles, lack of shivering, skin that feels ice cold, and a dead appearance. In addition to the previously discussed steps for treating a person with hypothermia, do the following:

1. Cut off the person's wet clothing.
2. Monitor the person's breathing; if absent, check the person's heart rate for 1 minute. If a heartbeat is not felt, give CPR and get an AED. **DO NOT** start CPR if any of the following scenarios exist:
   - The person has been submerged in cold water for more than 1 hour.
   - The person has obvious fatal injuries.
   - The person is frozen (eg, ice in the mouth and throat).
   - The person has a chest that is stiff or that cannot be compressed.

Heat-Related Emergencies

HEAT CRAMPS

Heat cramps are painful muscle spasms affecting the muscle in the back of the leg or abdomen that happen suddenly during or after physical exertion.

1. Have the person rest in a cool place.
2. Give lightly salted, cool water (dissolve one-fourth teaspoon [1.25 mL] salt in 1 quart [about 1 L] of water) or a commercial sports drink. **DO NOT** give salt tablets.

3. Stretch the cramped muscle or apply an ice pack for up to 20 minutes, placing a paper towel or thin cloth between the skin and the ice pack.

HEAT EXHAUSTION

Heat exhaustion differs from heatstroke because the person is alert and their skin may be clammy, not hot.

1. Move the person to a cool place.
2. Remove excess clothing.
3. Spray or douse cold water on the person's skin and vigorously fan the person.
4. If the person is able to swallow, give a commercial sports drink, fruit juice, or lightly salted water; if none of these options are available, give cold water. **DO NOT** give salt tablets.
5. Call 9-1-1 if improvement does not occur within 30 minutes. Heat exhaustion can turn into heatstroke.

HEATSTROKE

Heatstroke is life threatening and must be treated rapidly. The skin is extremely hot when touched and usually dry, but it may be wet from sweating related to strenuous work or exercise.

1. Call 9-1-1 as soon as possible.
2. Move the person to a cool place.
3. Remove clothing down to the person's underwear.
4. Cool the person quickly by any means possible, including any of the following methods (given in the order of effectiveness):
   a. Place the person in cold water, up to the neck. **DO NOT** leave the person alone.

b. Spray or douse cold water on the skin and vigorously fan the person.

c. Place ice packs against the person's armpits, groin, and sides of the neck.

Poison Ivy, Poison Oak, and Poison Sumac

WITHIN 5 MINUTES OF KNOWN CONTACT

1. Gently wipe skin with rubbing alcohol. **DO NOT** rub it in. **DO NOT** use packaged alcohol wipes. **DO NOT** use gasoline.

2. If rubbing alcohol is not available, wash the skin with a lot of cold running water. Soap is not necessary, but if used, rinse with a lot of cold running water. **DO NOT** scrub skin.

ITCHING AND MILD SWELLING

1. Apply any of the following:
   - Colloidal oatmeal bath (eg, Aveeno Soothing Bath Treatment)
   - Baking soda paste (made with 1 teaspoon [5 mL] water mixed with 3 teaspoons [15 mL] baking soda)
   - Calamine lotion
   - Physician-prescribed medication

2. If none of these are available, the application of OTC hydrocortisone may be beneficial.

SEVERE ITCHING, SWELLING, AND BLISTERS

1. Treat the same as for mild itching, or apply a physician-prescribed topical or oral steroid.

2. Seek professional medical care if the person inhaled smoke from a burning plant or if the reaction involves the face, eyes, genitals, or large areas of the body.

Poisoning

INHALED

All affected people require professional medical care even if they appear to have recovered.

1. Call 9-1-1 as soon as possible.
2. If the scene is not dangerous, immediately move the person into fresh air. If it appears unsafe, **DO NOT** enter the scene unless properly equipped and trained.
3. Monitor breathing; if absent, give CPR.
4. Try to determine the following:
   - What substance was inhaled?
   - When the exposure occurred?
   - How long the substance was inhaled?
   - The person's condition.
5. If the person is unresponsive and breathing, place the person on their side.

SWALLOWED

1. Try to determine:
   - Person's age and weight.
   - Person's condition.
   - What poison was swallowed?
   - When the poison was swallowed?
   - How much of the poison was swallowed?
2. If the person is responsive, call the Poison Control Center at 1-800-222-1222 and follow its directions (**FIGURE 15**).
3. If the person is unresponsive, call 9-1-1.

POISON Help
1-800-222-1222

FIGURE 15 If you or someone you know may have ingested a dangerous substance, contact poison control immediately at 1-800-222-1222 or go to poisonhelp .org for assistance.
Courtesy of the American Association of Poison Control Centers.

4. Place the person on their left side to delay the poison from moving into the intestines and to prevent inhalation of vomit, if it occurs.

5. Monitor breathing; if absent, call 9-1-1, if it has not been already done, and give CPR. Use a face shield or mask to avoid contact with vomit or poison.

6. *Cautions:*
   - **DO NOT** give anything to eat or drink unless advised to do so by the Poison Control Center.
   - **DO NOT** try to cause vomiting by giving syrup of ipecac or by gagging or tickling the back of the person's throat.
   - **DO NOT** give activated charcoal unless directed to do so by the Poison Control Center.
   - **DO NOT** follow the first aid procedures on a container's label because some have been known to be inaccurate.
   - **DO NOT** give water or milk to dilute poisons other than caustic or corrosive substances (acids and alkalis) unless told to do so by the Poison Control Center.

OPIOID OVERDOSE

Opioids include heroin and prescription pain medication (eg, morphine, oxycodone, hydrocodone). Any person who overdoses with an opioid requires professional medical care.

1. Check for breathing; if absent, give CPR. If a bystander is present, send the person to call 9-1-1 and to get an AED and naloxone while you give CPR. Naloxone can reverse the effects of an opioid overdose. Family members and friends of those known to be addicted to opioids may know if naloxone is available. If you are alone, give five sets of CPR before calling 9-1-1 and getting an AED and naloxone.

2. Give naloxone using one of the following methods:
   - Use a prefilled auto-injector. Inject naloxone by removing the cap to arm the syringe and pushing the syringe into the person's outer thigh.
   - Spray naloxone into a nostril using a nasal spray device.

3. If the person does not respond within 2 to 3 minutes, give another dose of naloxone. If the person is not breathing, continue giving CPR and using an AED, and administer another dose of naloxone.

NONOPIOID DRUG EMERGENCIES

1. If the person is alert and responsive, call the Poison Control Center at 1-800-222-1222.

2. If the person is unresponsive, call 9-1-1 and monitor breathing. If the person is not breathing, begin CPR.

CPR and AED

Adult and Child CPR and AED

Use the **RAB-CAB** mnemonic to remember what to do for a motionless person older than 1 year.

1. **R = Responsive?** Tap the person on the shoulder and shout, "Are you OK?" An unresponsive person will not react, answer, or move. Shout for nearby help.

2. **A = Activate** EMS and get an **AED**.
   - If you are alone and a mobile phone is available or a phone is nearby, call 9-1-1 with the speaker mode on.
   - If you are alone and a phone is not available, leave the person to locate a phone, call 9-1-1, and get an AED. For a child, give five sets of CPR before leaving them.
   - If a bystander is present and a mobile phone is available or a phone is nearby, ask the bystander to call 9-1-1 (with the speaker mode on) and get an AED while you give CPR.
   - If a bystander is present and a phone is not available, ask the bystander to go call 9-1-1 and get an AED while you give CPR.

3. **B = Breathing?** Check for no breathing or only occasional gasping.
   - Place the person faceup on a flat, firm surface.
   - Take 5 to 10 seconds to watch for chest movement.
   - If the person is not breathing or is only gasping (sounds similar to a quick inhalation or a snore, snort, or groan), continue to Step 4.

- If the person is breathing normally but not responding, CPR is not needed. Place the person on their side to keep the airway open.

4. **C = Compressions**.
   - Expose the person's chest by moving clothing out of the way.
   - Place the heel of one of your hands on the center of the person's chest (lower half of the breastbone; **FIGURE 16**).
   - For an adult or large child, place your other hand on top of the first, with your fingers interlocked.
   - Keep your arms straight and elbows locked, with your shoulders positioned directly over your hands.
   - Push hard and straight down on the breastbone, at least 2 inches (5 cm) for an adult, or about 2 inches (5 cm), or one-third the depth of the chest, for a child.

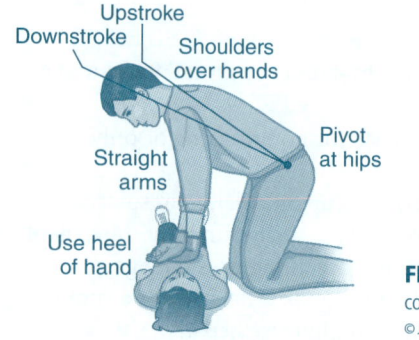

FIGURE 16 Chest compressions.
© Jones & Bartlett Learning.

- Push fast—100 to 120 compressions per minute. Consider using the beat of the Bee Gees song "Stayin' Alive", the beats from a smartphone app that was previously installed and is quickly accessible, or a dispatcher's directions heard over a cell phone's speaker.
- Allow the chest to rise fully after each compression. **DO NOT** lean or bounce on the chest.

5. **A = Airway**. Open the person's airway, using the head tilt–chin lift (**FIGURE 17**).

6. **B = Breaths**.
   - Pinch the person's nose shut. With your mouth, make an airtight mouth-to-mouth seal; use a CPR mask or face shield if available.
   - Give 2 breaths, each lasting 1 second, to make the chest rise.
   - If breaths do not cause the person's chest to rise, begin CPR. Each time before giving a set of breaths, open the mouth and look for an object; if one is seen, remove it.

7. Use an AED as soon as possible.
   - Turn on the AED and follow its prompts.

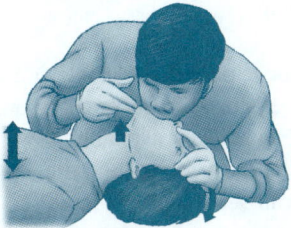

FIGURE 17 To give rescue breaths, open the person's airway using the head tilt–chin lift maneuver.
© Jones & Bartlett Learning.

- Attach the pads to the person's bare, dry chest (as shown on the pads' diagrams). For a child, use child-sized pads if available.
- Make sure that no one is touching the person. Say, "Clear!"
- Allow the AED to analyze the person's heart rhythm. The AED will prompt one of two actions:
  - Stay clear and press the shock button to deliver a shock.
  - Shock is not needed; resume CPR. Pads can remain in place.
- After performing any one of the actions, give CPR until the AED prompts another heart analysis (ie, every 2 minutes).

8. Continue performing CPR and using the AED until one of the following occurs:
   - The person moves, reacts, or begins breathing.
   - EMS or another trained person takes over.

Infant CPR

Use the **RAB-CAB** mnemonic to remember what to do.

1. **R = Responsive?** Tap the infant's foot and shout their name. Shout for nearby help.
2. **A = Activate** EMS.
   - If you are alone and a mobile phone is available or a phone is nearby, call 9-1-1 with the speaker mode on.
   - If you are alone and a phone is not available, give five sets of CPR. Then, while carrying the infant, locate a phone, call 9-1-1, and get an AED. Continue giving CPR.

- If a bystander is present and a mobile phone is available or a phone is nearby, ask the person to call 9-1-1 (with the speaker mode on) and to get an AED while you give CPR.
- If a bystander is present and a phone is not available, ask the bystander to locate a phone, call 9-1-1, and get an AED while you give CPR.

3. **B = Breathing?** Place the infant faceup on an elevated flat, firm surface (eg, table, cabinet top). Take 5 to 10 seconds to watch from neck to waist for movement.

4. **C = Compressions**.

   Single rescuers can use either the encircling thumbs technique or the two-finger technique. If the rescuer cannot physically encircle the infant's chest, use the two-finger technique.

   - To perform the encircling thumbs technique, do the following:
     a. Expose the infant's chest by moving clothing out of the way.
     b. Place both thumbs on the lower third of the breastbone, both touching the imaginary nipple line and the fingers encircling the infant's back and chest (**FIGURE 18**).

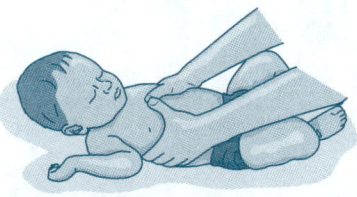

FIGURE 18 Encircling thumbs technique for an infant.
© Jones & Bartlett Learning.

   c. Give 30 chest compressions. Push hard and straight down, about 1.5 inches (4 cm), or at least one-third the depth of the chest. Push fast (consider using the beat of the Bee Gees song "Stayin' Alive", the beats from a smartphone app that was previously installed and is quickly accessible, or a dispatcher's directions heard over a cell phone's speaker).

   d. Allow the chest to rise fully after each compression.

- To perform the two-finger technique, do the following:

   a. Expose the infant's chest by moving clothing out of the way.

   b. Place the pads of two fingers on the infant's breastbone (center of chest), with one touching and both below the nipple line (**FIGURE 19**).

   c. Give 30 chest compressions. Push hard and fast as described for the encircling thumbs technique.

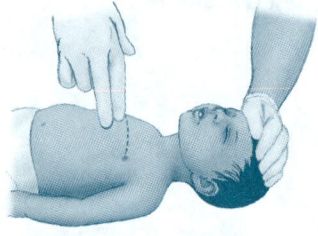

FIGURE 19 Two-finger compression technique for an infant.
© Jones & Bartlett Learning.

   d. Allow the chest to rise fully after each
       compression.
5. **A = Airway**. Perform the head tilt–chin lift, with one
   hand on the infant's forehead and one or two fingers
   of the other hand on the bony part of the jaw.
6. **B = Breaths**. With your mouth, make an airtight
   mouth-to-mouth and nose seal. If this does not
   work, try either mouth-to-mouth or mouth-to-nose
   breaths. Use a CPR mask or face shield if available.
   Give 2 breaths, each lasting 1 second, to make the
   infant's chest rise (**FIGURE 20**).
7. Continue CPR until one of the following occurs:
   - The infant begins breathing.
   - EMS arrives and takes over.
   - You become physically exhausted and unable to
     continue.
8. If another person is available, trade off about every
   five sets of CPR (2 minutes).

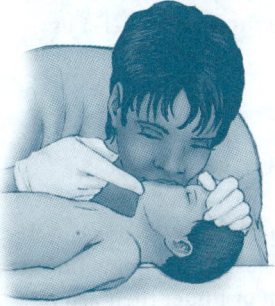

FIGURE 20 Give CPR to an infant
with your mouth over the infant's
mouth and nose.
© Jones & Bartlett Learning.

Compression-Only CPR

If you are not trained in CPR or you are unable or unwilling to make mouth-to-mouth contact, give compression-only CPR.

1. Ask another person to call 9-1-1.
2. Place the person on a firm, flat surface.
3. Push the center of the chest hard and fast (to the beat of the Bee Gees song "Stayin' Alive", the beats from a smartphone app that was previously installed and is quickly accessible, or a dispatcher's directions heard over a cell phone's speaker).
4. Continue chest compression without stopping until help arrives, or as long as possible. If another person is available, trade off about every 2 minutes.

Airway Obstruction and Choking Care

A combination of back blows and abdominal thrusts (5 back blows followed by 5 abdominal thrusts, known as the 5 and 5 approach) should be used to dislodge an airway obstruction (choking). Airway obstruction can be life-threatening, so call 9-1-1 as soon as possible.

BACK BLOWS

1. Ask, "Are you choking?" or "Do you need help?" Shout for nearby help to alert others of the emergency.
2. Stand behind the person and slightly to one side. Reach across the person's chest by wrapping one arm either over the person's arm or under their armpit.

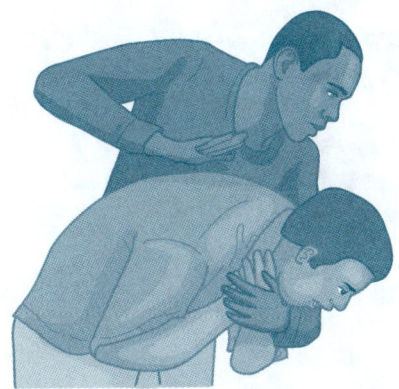

FIGURE 21 Back blows for choking care.
© Jones & Bartlett Learning.

Place the palm of that hand on the person's upper chest or shoulder. Leave your other hand free.

3. Have the person bend over at the waist to a 90° angle.

4. With your fingertips up, use the heel of your hand to firmly strike the person between their shoulder blades (**FIGURE 21**). **DO NOT** just pat them on the back. Use hard blows, like driving a nail into a thick board with a hammer.

5. If 5 back blows do not dislodge the object, give up to 5 abdominal thrusts.

ABDOMINAL THRUSTS

1. Ask, "Are you choking?" or "Do you need help?" Shout for nearby help to alert others of the emergency.

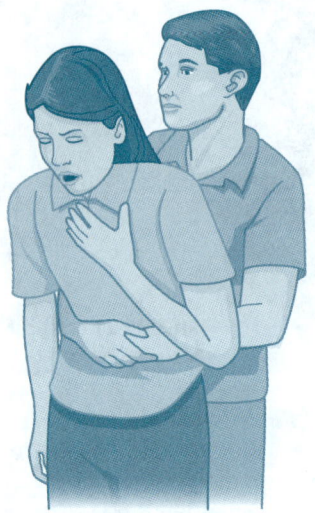

FIGURE 22 Stand behind the person and wrap your arms around their waist.
© Jones & Bartlett Learning.

2. Stand behind an adult; stand or kneel behind a child. Put one foot between the person's feet for balance. If the person is a lot taller than you, have them kneel or sit in front of you. Wrap your arms around the person's waist (**FIGURE 22**). Locate the person's navel with one finger.

3. Make a fist with the other hand and place the thumb side of this hand just above the person's navel and below the tip of the breastbone.

4. Grasp the fist with the other hand. Thrust the fist into the person's abdomen with a quick upward motion. Use chest thrusts on a person who is choking and obese or pregnant. Each thrust should

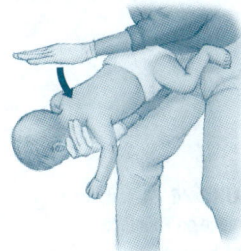

FIGURE 23 Back blow technique on an infant.
© Jones & Bartlett Learning.

be a separate and distinct effort to dislodge the object. Continue without interruption until the person coughs up the object, speaks, or breathes.

UNRESPONSIVE ADULT AND CHILD CHOKING

1. Give 30 chest compressions.
2. Give 2 breaths.
3. Continue sets of 30 chest compressions and 2 breaths. Each time before giving the first of the 2 breaths, look into the mouth for an object; if one is seen, remove it.

RESPONSIVE INFANT CHOKING

1. Give up to 5 separate and distinct back blows as follows (**FIGURE 23**):
   a. Support the infant's head with your hand.
   b. Lay the infant facedown over your forearm, with the head lower than their chest.
   c. Brace your forearm and the infant against your thigh.

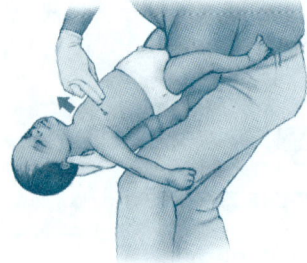

FIGURE 24 Chest thrust technique on an infant.
© Jones & Bartlett Learning.

    d. Give the back blows between the infant's shoulder blades with the heel of your other hand.
    e. If the object does not come out, turn the infant onto their back while supporting the head.

2. Give up to 5 separate and distinct chest thrusts as follows (**FIGURE 24**):
    a. Support the infant's head with your hand.
    b. Lay the infant faceup over your forearm, with the head lower than their chest.
    c. Brace your forearm and the infant against your thigh.
    d. Place two fingers of your other hand in the same location as for giving CPR compressions.
    e. Give the thrusts 1 second apart; these thrusts are not as fast as CPR compressions.

3. Continue alternating the 5 back blows and 5 chest thrusts without interruption until the infant stops responding or can breathe, cough, or cry.

UNRESPONSIVE INFANT CHOKING

1. Give 30 chest compressions.
2. Give 2 breaths.
3. Continue sets of 30 chest compressions and 2 breaths. Each time before giving the first of the 2 breaths, look into the mouth for an object; if one is seen, remove it.

Emergency Telephone Numbers and Information

Local Emergency Number (Usually 9-1-1): ....

On-site Emergency Response Number: ....

Poison Control Center: **1-800-222-1222**

National Suicide Prevention Lifeline: **9-8-8**

Physician's Name and Number: ....

Neighbor's Name and Number: ....

Relative's Name and Number: ....

Your Home/Residence

Address: ....

....

....

Telephone Number: ....

Nearest Intersection or Landmark: ....

Emergency Equipment and Supplies Locations

First Aid Kit Location: ....

AED Location: ....

Quick Emergency Index